Sharing Wellness Info:

Ready

for Health Care Emergencies

Dedication

To those whose lives may be saved by being prepared
and having their family, friends, and agents prepared.
May your lives be blessed with eternal good health.

Sharing Wellness Info:
Ready
for Health Care Emergencies

Gail Coffey

www.SharingWellnessInfo.com

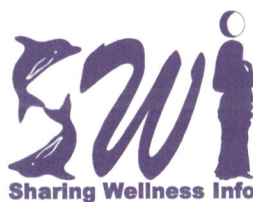

Sharing Wellness Info

ceo@sharingwellnessinfo.com or cio@sharingwellnessinfo.com

3210 Ravensworth Place

Alexandria, VA 22302

www.sharingwellnessinfo.com

ISBN-13: 978-0-6151-4268-5

ISBN-10: 0-61514268-5

Library of Congress Catalog Number: requested 02/07

Printed in the United States

Acknowledgements With Deep Appreciation

I wish to acknowledge and thank John Coffey for his willingness to be the "star" or reason for this article and permission to use his actual name. Thank you to several people who provided editorial support and encouragement to publish this piece: Mary Ludwig, Laura Abramson, Charlotte Hayes, Linda MacDonald, Lyndy Pacheco, Reva Wine, Jen Power, and Anne Strozier-Adams (as well as their friends and family members). Without their encouragement, this would never have been published.

Thank you to Angela K. Ludwig for the cover design and formatting of this document for publication.

Table of Contents

Sharing Wellness Info: Ready for Health Care Emergencies

By Gail Coffey, CEO of SharingWellnessInfo.com

Be Prepared—The Life You Save Could Be Your Own!

In a medical emergency would your friends, housemates, spouses, children, or other emergency contact(s) have the information that could save your life?

Emergencies happen and can happen to you -- or to someone who has listed you as an emergency contact -- or to someone with whom you share living or work space.

Give Your Emergency Plan a Reality Check

Have you considered how an emergency contact of yours would access you? Do they have to get through security? Do they have a key to your home in case you are not able to admit them? Do they have instructions that include your physician's name, address, telephone number; your hospital of choice? Do you carry this contact's information on you in case you are found unconscious for any reason—or unable to speak? Does your health care representative know about any allergies you have? Do they know what kind of care you want to have in life-threatening situations? Have you identified a medical durable power of attorney in case you are unconscious and medical decisions have to be made? If so, does your emergency contact (and/or relevant friends and family members) have a copy? These questions came to my mind because of a phone call I received recently and succeeding events that unfolded.

The Phone Call

One quiet Wednesday afternoon I received a phone call that turned my life topsy-turvy for a few weeks. With this call I became aware of how little essential information is available should people around me need to help in a medical emergency. I'm fairly organized; I've done a "what my family should know" document and sent it to my son and daughter who live within a 50-mile radius of me—a year ago. I've told them where to find legal documents they might need in case of my death or a coma. But one result of that 3:30pm Wednesday phone call is that I realized my friends, who live within my same apartment building or within less than a 10-mile radius—and who might be the first ones to help me in a medical emergency, had none of that information and that none of them—friends or family—had all the information they would need in a true medical emergency.

When Sudden Illness Comes to Call

So, how did this Wednesday afternoon phone call I received make such a big impression on me?

My ex-husband, John, and I generally see or talk to each other about 3 or 4 times a year, usually at family gatherings. I became aware of being listed as his emergency contact at his work by receiving a call from them requesting my help in obtaining his cell phone number. I gave them the number—and promptly forgot all about being listed as his emergency contact.

This Wednesday afternoon phone call was much different. A woman from his office told me John had been taken to an emergency room the previous day. Two people from his office had spoken to him during this Wednesday, and John did not sound "like himself." She was requesting that I "lay eyes on him" and report back to them as to whether John was okay.

Because I knew of a heart bypass that John had undergone 6 years earlier, I asked if the emergency room visit had been due to a heart event. I was told that it was severe lower back pain—to the point of near inability to walk.

Stranger and Stranger

With a degree in health theology and many years of study regarding health issues, severe lower back pain did not equate to someone's "not sounding like oneself" and I wondered what information was missing and I began to realize how little I knew about any health concerns of John's since the fall of 2001.

There were several potential challenges to "laying eyes on him." As I explained to the caller, John lives in a secure complex. I would need to call him to see if he would agree to "ring me in" to his building and to his apartment. If he were unable to answer the phone, I would need to be on an admissions list to use his courtesy key. If I was not on such a list, I would have to convince the condo's security personnel to escort me to his door. Life can be so complicated! And, with sickness, it becomes even more so.

I called both John's home and cell phone numbers and got voice mail on both. I called the condominium office and learned that I was listed as an emergency contact but not on the admissions list. I explained the call I had just received and asked if security could escort me to his condo and eventually, security agreed to do so.

I met the security guard. We proceeded to John's building where the guard provided admittance; then to John's door, where the guard knocked and knocked and knocked and rang the bell and rang the bell and knocked some more. As the guard pondered what to do next, we heard a voice saying something from inside. (Approximately 30 to 40 minutes had now elapsed since receiving the phone call. Had this been a stroke or heart attack, he could have died in this amount of time.)

John opened the door, wearing a bathrobe, and looking intently at the guard who was asking John if he needed help, did he need him to call 911, was he okay? John didn't respond with words or a look that seemed to comprehend the questions. Finally, I repeated the "are you okay" question and he swung his head to look at me. His face showed some kind of recognition, but he still didn't answer the question. He was swaying a little and was holding himself upright by leaning against the top of the door casing. I asked him if he needed to sit down.

John said "probably," the first word we had heard. I then asked if we might enter and he backed up so we could do so and started for a chair. After getting a swallow of water, he sat down.

The guard told me he thought he was no longer needed unless I wanted him to call 911. Since I was still trying to assess what was going on, I said it was okay for the guard to leave.

I asked John a number of questions and he tried to answer. He would look at me; he would start to say something and then, as if his speech ability was stuck and he would begin to say "er, er, er, er" and get frustrated. He showed no signs of visible paralysis; his color appeared normal.

Really Sick People Don't Answer Questions Well

I questioned John, looking for clues to what was going on. Had he taken some medicine that was causing this? Had he gotten confused during the night and taken an extra dose of pain medication? His color looked fairly normal, but he couldn't seem to answer me consistently as to whether he had pain. Sometimes he said yes and sometimes he said no. Finally, I began to look around to see if I could see pill bottles or a PDA with his doctor's information.

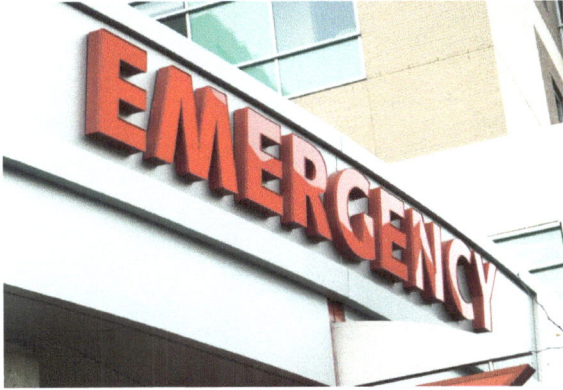

I saw papers from a hospital lying on a table near the front door. Although the papers gave no hospital address, they provided the date and time of the visit from the night before. He had been diagnosed with back pain from what they believed to be a muscular cause. The papers listed the drugs that had been prescribed. I found no pill bottles with those drugs in them either on the table, in his kitchen, his bathroom, or by his bed.

More Confusion and Worry

In the search for the prescriptions, I went to his bathroom and found an older and different prescription bottle with a doctor's name. I asked him if that were his doctor. He confirmed this and repeated the doctor's name a couple of times. I had to call information to get the doctor's number. I called the doctor's office and described the situation. They told me to take him directly to an emergency room as it could be a stroke or any of a number of other serious disorders.

I told John I thought I should call 911. He refused. (In hindsight, I now realize that listening to an otherwise incoherent person was not wise and could have caused significant problems—delay in getting him to medical care; he could have fallen or gotten hurt as I steered him by the elbow to the car, etc.) I helped him into clothing I found on the bedroom floor, apparently dropped there the night before, sandals, and a jacket that was by the table in his living room.

I found some insurance cards and credit cards in a holder on the table with the hospital emergency room papers. I collected the cards (hoping they contained his health insurance information) his keys, and his money clip. I got him into his car (the nearest one) and drove him to the nearest emergency room that I knew.

Short Term Memory Gone at the Worst Possible Time

At the emergency room, John was unable to give his name; but was able to give his social security number and his date of birth. He was otherwise unable to answer any questions about his health or about the ER visit the previous day. He could tell the hospital personnel nothing except his social security number and, sometimes, his date of birth.

As it turned out, the cards I had picked up had no driver's license to validate his identity and no health insurance card. I was not able to provide the recent health history information his medical team needed. I couldn't say whether he had any known allergies; what medications he had taken; or what medications he was on routinely.

I called John's office associate to let her know John's condition, that he was at the Emergency Care Facility, and that the hospital needed insurance information. She was able to give me the insurance company name and group number but could not provide John's individual number. She gave me a human resources number. When I called the following day, they would not provide the number to me and would not confirm whether they would contact the hospital with the number.

By this time, I was beginning to realize the precarious position both John and I were in: he could not communicate; his life might be at stake; I had no legal standing with anyone regarding his care—no authority; and I had very little information. I had no idea how John wanted to be treated, by whom, or to what extent. I began to wonder what if he didn't regain the ability to speak? What if he had someone designated to be his medical power of attorney? What if he needed very serious medical procedures?

Answers and More Questions

John was not fully able to participate and respond with details of his own medical history for 48 to 72 hours. During this time he was diagnosed with delirium from a very high fever caused by methicillin resistant staph aureus (MRSA). A week later, he was taken into surgery to drain an abscess on the lower lumbar area of his spinal column that was the result of the infection.

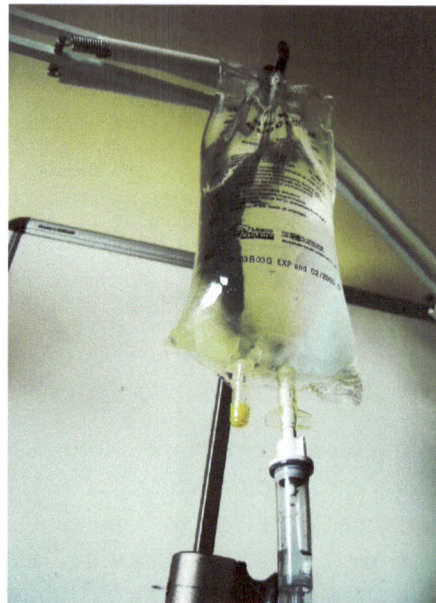

For several hours, John had not been able to provide any information about his own state of being. For several days, he was not clear about many details of current or past health events, or where to find the information required.

As John became more cogent, he contacted friends, relatives and co-workers with his cell phone, but found he had very limited energy to talk and had a hard time keeping straight all that was happening to him. I stayed with him as much as possible, functioning as memory and voice and monitoring his care. I allowed our same last name to facilitate obtaining information on his behalf, repeating it over and over so he could ingest the information and process it slowly. I acted as his health care advocate. When not at the hospital I researched information about what he was being told, emailed reports of his progress to an email group to keep calls to a minimum, and kept his management team at work up to date. Gradually he became able to update his own medical history for the medical team and involved some of his other friends and co-workers as his support team.

Information is Critical in An Emergency

John was hospitalized for a total of 14 days; had all kinds of tests including a spinal tap done in the emergency room; the surgery to drain the abscess; preliminary diagnoses that ranged from pneumonia to endocarditis and then the possibility of staph aureus on his heart valves. Because of the resistance to antibiotics and the adaptability that staph aureus has shown to mutate to varieties that continue to resist new antibiotics, John was sent home after 14 days to continue IV antibiotics for at least 6 weeks; with simultaneous oral antibiotic that will have to continue even after the IV treatment is discontinued.

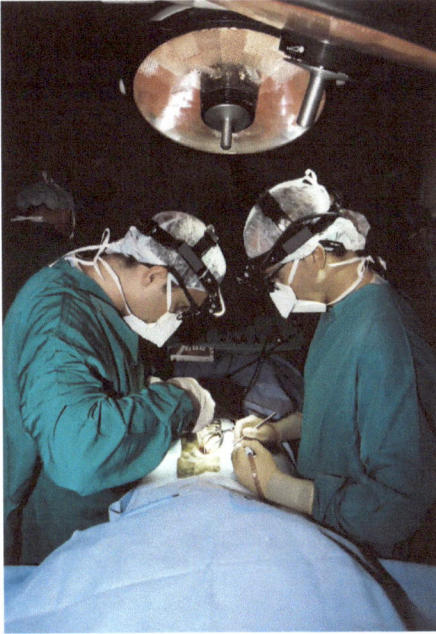

John did not have an advance medical directive or a living will (see definitions and information that follow in this article). I had no information to help his medical team make a faster diagnosis.

This experience made me realize that those most likely to need similar information should I have a medical emergency also didn't have such information that could save my life—and was the genesis of this article.

Like many, John and I are both intelligent, educated, and fairly well-informed individuals regarding medical issues. Yet neither of us had realized the significance of the term "emergency contact." I hope sharing this experience will benefit *you*.

What You Can Do to Avoid a Situation Like John's

I've put together a checklist for you, based on these recent lessons learned. The checklist applies to you and to anyone for whom you may the support and/or advocate regarding health/wellness.

Whether you are naming someone as your emergency contact or being named, be sure that the appropriate information is shared BEFORE it is required in a medical emergency.

The information needs to be updated *at least once a year*. Email is a great way to distribute it, or just drop copies in the mail to close family and friends. There must be a directive that has been witnessed or notarized (per your state's requirements) with this information in order for you to represent the person who has designated you as emergency contact if you have no legally recognized relationship to the person. This is *especially* true if designating a friend rather than a relative or spouse to be your representative.

Basic Health Information for Emergency Contact, Friends, Family		

Full Name:		

Street Address:		Apt. #
City:	State:	Zip Code:
SSN:	Blood Type:	
Date of Birth:	Place of Birth:	

Gen. Practitioner's Name and Practice Address:	
GP's phone #:	

Insurance Information

Company name:	Individual member #:	Group #:
	Address of Ins. Co.:	Ins. Phone #:

Secondary health insurance:

Company name:	Individual member #:	Group #:
	Address of Ins. Co.:	Phone #:
Medicare Info:		
Allergies (food/drugs/chemicals):		
Sensitivities (foods/drugs/etc):		

History of surgeries:

Name of Surgery	Date	Location & Doc's Name

Basic Health Information for Emergency Contact, Friends, Family		

Other Important Information:	
Advance Directive? Location:	
Contact info for durable medical power of attorney:	
Living Will? Location:	
Contact info for durable medical power of attorney:	
Will? Location?	
Attorney's contact info: Point of Contact:	

Friends/Family contacts:		
Person	**Relationship** (parent, child, sibling, friend)	**Email/phone #**

Work Contacts:		
Person	**Title**	**Email/phone #**
	Boss	
	Human Resources	

Basic Health Information
for Emergency Contact, Friends, Family

Ongoing health problems:

Problem	Onset	Treatment:

Medications taken daily or regularly:

Name	Dosage/frequency	Name of prescribing doctor

Be Prepared – the Life You Save May be Your Own!

Don't let yourself be caught without your friends, housemates, spouses, children, or other emergency contact(s) having the information that could save your life. Emergencies happen and some emergency could happen to you! Or to someone who has put you down as an emergency contact--or to someone with whom you share living or work space.

Suggestions for Keeping Information Current and Available

Keep your wallet card with your insurance card so they will be found together. This will make it easier for you to remember. The wallet card is a small "cheat sheet" for you in an emergency situation when it's hard to remember the kinds of information needed—and easier than fumbling through your PDA, address book, looking for business cards, or checking your phone for numbers.

Put an SWI info reminder on your birthday on your annual calendar, your computer reminders, and anywhere else that will remind you to update the information at least once a year.

Make Important Decisions While You are Well

Do you have an advance directive, a living will, or have you completed the Five Wishes documentation?

If just reading the words "advance directive" or "living will" causes you to freeze up, then try reading through the Five Wishes web site (link at end of this article). In many ways, this organization helps walk you through the process for stating the care you want to have with compassion and leads you to compile complete information that anyone caring for you in an emergency might need.

Completing the Five Wishes documentation means that *you* specify the person you want to make medical care decisions for you when you cannot; *you* specify the kind of medical treatment you want or do not want; *you* specify how comfortable you want to be; *you* specify how you want people to treat you; and what *you* want your loved ones to know. In many states this document can be used in place of advance directives and/or living wills—check with your local (state) authorities or attorney.

An Advance Directive lets other people know the types of medical care you do and do not want in the event you are unable to express your wishes on your own. In Virginia, there are two kinds of Advance Directives: 1) appointment of an agent (medical power of attorney) and 2) a living will.

You may also state what kinds of life-prolonging treatment you want or do not want if you are diagnosed as having a terminal condition and you are unable to express your own wishes. The legal term for this is a "living will."

There is no national standard in the United States for health care directives; to ensure that your wishes are followed, you must consult state representatives or an attorney to comply with your state regulations. The Five Wishes is accepted in 38 states at the time of this writing.

➤ The Five Wishes documentation can be obtained from
http://www.agingwithdignity.org/5wishes.html.

Advance Directives are different for each State within the United States. Samples of forms for each state can be found at Caring Connections:

➤ http://www.caringinfo.org/i4a/pages/Index.cfm?pageid=3425.

Psychiatric Advance Directive information can be found at:

➤ http://www.bazelon.org/issues/advancedirectives/index.htm

Be sure to have the form legally reviewed for its durability and legality in your own state.

Commonwealth of Virginia information on advance directives, living wills, etc. within the commonwealth:

➤ http://www.vsb.org/publications/brochure/health.html

Virginia Department of Aging sample medical directive and living will forms that work in the Commonwealth of Virginia:

➤   http://www.aging.state.va.us/pdfdocs/AdvMedDir.pdf

Sample living will and durable medical power of attorney from Georgetown (check the viability of these forms with regard to your own state's requirements):

➤   http://www.georgetown.edu/research/nrcbl/publications/scopenotes/sn2.pdf

The Virginia State Bar provides a sample advance directive/living form on their site:

➤   http://www.vsb.org/sections/hl/add06/2005Form.pdf

There are also organizations that sell these forms such as LegacyWriter.com where the cost is $20.00. Because each state varies so much, I recommend having a local attorney review whatever you put together for its viability in your area.

➤   http://www.legacywriter.com/livingwill.asp?src=g12healthcaredirectivesd

Another excellent form to help you pull together all of your information that family and/or friends might need to know is available from the Washington National Guard at

➤   http://familysupport.washingtonguard.com/NewsLetters/Spt_Files/What_My_Family_Should_Know. pdf.

Copies of this article may be downloaded from the member only section of *www.sharingwellnessinfo.com* (wellness tools area) or requested by writing to: info@sharingwellnessinfo.com

Check List for Your Notebook

These are suggestions of emergency information for inclusion in your notebook or folder. You may wish to keep one notebook/file for everyone—or a notebook for each person for whom you have any responsibility, so that it is easy to grab only what you need.

For You

_____ My own Emergency Medical Contacts

_____ My Advance Directive/Living Will or Five Wishes forms completed and signed

_____ My wallet card completed and in my wallet/purse

_____ What My Family Needs to Know forms completed (financial data, will, other records)

For Family Members

_____ Emergency Medical Contact form completed for spouse/lover

_____ Wallet card completed and in wallet/purse for spouse/lover

_____ Advance Directive/Living Will or Five Wishes forms completed and signed for spouse/lover

_____ Emergency Medical Contact form completed for son

_____ Wallet card completed and in wallet/purse for son

_____ Advance Directive/Living Will or Five Wishes forms completed and signed for son

_____ Emergency Medical Contact form completed for daughter

_____ Wallet card completed and in wallet/purse for daughter

_____ Advance Directive/Living Will or Five Wishes forms completed and signed for daughter

_____ Emergency Medical Contact form completed for parent

_____ Wallet card completed and in wallet/purse for parent

_____ Advance Directive/Living Will or Five Wishes forms completed and signed for parent

_____ Emergency Medical Contact form completed for parent

_____

Wallet card completed and in wallet/purse for parent

_____

Advance Directive/Living Will or Five Wishes forms completed and signed for parent

_____

Emergency Medical Contact form completed for other

_____

Wallet card completed and in wallet/purse for other

_____

Advance Directive/Living Will or Five Wishes forms completed and signed for other

_____

Extra Emergency Contact Sheets

Basic Health Information for Emergency Contact, Friends, Family		
Full Name:		
Street Address:		Apt. #
City:	State:	Zip Code:
SSN:	Blood Type:	
Date of Birth:	Place of Birth:	
Gen. Practitioner's Name and Practice Address:		
GP's phone #:		
Insurance Information		
Company name:	Individual member #:	Group #:
	Address of Ins. Co.:	Ins. Phone #:
Secondary health insurance:		
Company name:	Individual member #:	Group #:
	Address of Ins. Co.:	Phone #:
Medicare Info:		
Allergies (food/drugs/ chemicals):		
Sensitivities (foods/ drugs/etc):		

Are You Prepared for Health Care Emergencies?

Basic Health Information for Emergency Contact, Friends, Family

History of surgeries:

Name of Surgery	Date	Location & Doc's Name

Other Important Information:

Advance Directive? Location:	
Contact info for durable medical power of attorney:	
Living Will? Location:	
Contact info for durable medical power of attorney:	
Will? Location?	
Attorney's contact info: Point of Contact:	

Friends/Family contacts:

Person	Relationship (parent, child, sibling, friend)	Email/phone #

Are You Prepared for Health Care Emergencies?

Basic Health Information
for Emergency Contact, Friends, Family

Work Contacts:

Person	Title	Email/phone #
	Boss	
	Human Resources	

Ongoing health problems:

Problem	Onset	Treatment:

Medications taken daily or regularly:

Name	Dosage/frequency	Name of prescribing doctor

Basic Health Information
for Emergency Contact, Friends, Family

Full Name:		
Street Address:		**Apt. #**
City:	**State:**	**Zip Code:**
SSN:	**Blood Type:**	
Date of Birth:	**Place of Birth:**	
Gen. Practitioner's Name and Practice Address:		
GP's phone #:		

Insurance Information

Company name:	Individual member #:	Group #:
	Address of Ins. Co.:	Ins. Phone #:

Secondary health insurance:

Company name:	Individual member #:	Group #:
	Address of Ins. Co.:	Phone #:
Medicare Info:		
Allergies (food/drugs/ chemicals):		
Sensitivities (foods/ drugs/etc):		

Basic Health Information
for Emergency Contact, Friends, Family

History of surgeries:

Name of Surgery	Date	Location & Doc's Name

Other Important Information:

Advance Directive? Location:	
Contact info for durable medical power of attorney:	
Living Will? Location:	
Contact info for durable medical power of attorney:	
Will? Location?	
Attorney's contact info: Point of Contact:	

Friends/Family contacts:

Person	Relationship (parent, child, sibling, friend)	Email/phone #

Basic Health Information
for Emergency Contact, Friends, Family

Work Contacts:

Person	Title	Email/phone #
	Boss	
	Human Resources	

Ongoing health problems:

Problem	Onset	Treatment:

Medications taken daily or regularly:

Name	Dosage/frequency	Name of prescribing doctor

Basic Health Information
for Emergency Contact, Friends, Family

Full Name:		
Street Address:		Apt. #
City:	State:	Zip Code:
SSN:	Blood Type:	
Date of Birth:	Place of Birth:	
Gen. Practitioner's Name and Practice Address:		
GP's phone #:		

Insurance Information

Company name:	Individual member #:	Group #:
	Address of Ins. Co.:	Ins. Phone #:

Secondary health insurance:

Company name:	Individual member #:	Group #:
	Address of Ins. Co.:	Phone #:
Medicare Info:		
Allergies (food/drugs/chemicals):		
Sensitivities (foods/drugs/etc):		

Basic Health Information
for Emergency Contact, Friends, Family

History of surgeries:

Name of Surgery	Date	Location & Doc's Name

Other Important Information:

Advance Directive? Location:	
Contact info for durable medical power of attorney:	
Living Will? Location:	
Contact info for durable medical power of attorney:	
Will? Location?	
Attorney's contact info: Point of Contact:	

Friends/Family contacts:

Person	Relationship (parent, child, sibling, friend)	Email/phone #

Basic Health Information
for Emergency Contact, Friends, Family

Work Contacts:

Person	Title	Email/phone #
	Boss	
	Human Resources	

Ongoing health problems:

Problem	Onset	Treatment:

Medications taken daily or regularly:

Name	Dosage/frequency	Name of prescribing doctor

Basic Health Information
for Emergency Contact, Friends, Family

Full Name:		
Street Address:		**Apt. #**
City:	**State:**	**Zip Code:**
SSN:	**Blood Type:**	
Date of Birth:	**Place of Birth:**	

Gen. Practitioner's Name and Practice Address:	
GP's phone #:	

Insurance Information

Company name:	Individual member #:	Group #:
	Address of Ins. Co.:	Ins. Phone #:

Secondary health insurance:

Company name:	Individual member #:	Group #:
	Address of Ins. Co.:	Phone #:
Medicare Info:		
Allergies (food/drugs/ chemicals):		
Sensitivities (foods/ drugs/etc):		

Basic Health Information
for Emergency Contact, Friends, Family

History of surgeries:

Name of Surgery	Date	Location & Doc's Name

Other Important Information:

Advance Directive? Location:	
Contact info for durable medical power of attorney:	
Living Will? Location:	
Contact info for durable medical power of attorney:	
Will? Location?	
Attorney's contact info: Point of Contact:	

Friends/Family contacts:

Person	Relationship (parent, child, sibling, friend)	Email/phone #

Basic Health Information
for Emergency Contact, Friends, Family

Work Contacts:

Person	Title	Email/phone #
	Boss	
	Human Resources	

Ongoing health problems:

Problem	Onset	Treatment:

Medications taken daily or regularly:

Name	Dosage/frequency	Name of prescribing doctor

Basic Health Information
for Emergency Contact, Friends, Family

Full Name:	

Street Address:		Apt. #

City:	State:	Zip Code:

SSN:	Blood Type:

Date of Birth:	Place of Birth:

Gen. Practitioner's Name and Practice Address:	
GP's phone #:	

Insurance Information

Company name:	Individual member #:	Group #:
	Address of Ins. Co.:	Ins. Phone #:

Secondary health insurance:

Company name:	Individual member #:	Group #:
	Address of Ins. Co.:	Phone #:
Medicare Info:		
Allergies (food/drugs/ chemicals):		
Sensitivities (foods/ drugs/etc):		

Are You Prepared for Health Care Emergencies?

Basic Health Information
for Emergency Contact, Friends, Family

History of surgeries:

Name of Surgery	Date	Location & Doc's Name

Other Important Information:

Advance Directive? Location:	
Contact info for durable medical power of attorney:	
Living Will? Location:	
Contact info for durable medical power of attorney:	
Will? Location?	
Attorney's contact info: Point of Contact:	

Friends/Family contacts:

Person	Relationship (parent, child, sibling, friend)	Email/phone #

Basic Health Information
for Emergency Contact, Friends, Family

Work Contacts:

Person	Title	Email/phone #
	Boss	
	Human Resources	

Ongoing health problems:

Problem	Onset	Treatment:

Medications taken daily or regularly:

Name	Dosage/frequency	Name of prescribing doctor

Wallet Cards

Attention Medical Personnel: I have an Advance Directive/Living Will.

_____
Signature

Please consult my document and/or my Power of Attorney in an emergency. My representative is:

Name _____

Address _____

Phone _____

Attention Medical Personnel: My blood type _____.

My allergies:_____ _____

Daily Medications: _____

_____

Epileptic__ Diabetic__ Asthma__ Other_____

Primary Care Physician _____

Phone _____

Attention Medical Personnel:

Contacts to obtain a copy of my Advance Directive.

_____
Name of Agent/Durable Medical Power of Attorney

_____
Phone

Name of Alternative Agent/Durable Medical Power of Attorney

_____
Phone

_____
Name
        Phone

Attention Medical Personnel:

My name: _____

SSN or D/L _____ DOB _____

Insurance Carrier & Number _____

Place of Business _____

Business Contact Phone such as boss _____

Other Info _____

Attention Medical Personnel: I have an Advance Directive/Living Will.

_____
Signature

Please consult my document and/or my Power of Attorney in an emergency. My representative is:

Name _____

Address _____

Phone _____

Attention Medical Personnel: My blood type _____.

My allergies:_____ _____

Daily Medications: _____

_____

Epileptic__ Diabetic__ Asthma__ Other_____

Primary Care Physician _____

Phone _____

Attention Medical Personnel:

Contacts to obtain a copy of my Advance Directive.

_____
Name of Agent/Durable Medical Power of Attorney

_____
Phone

Name of Alternative Agent/Durable Medical Power of Attorney

_____
Phone

_____
Name
        Phone

Attention Medical Personnel:

My name: _____

SSN or D/L _____ DOB _____

Insurance Carrier & Number _____

Place of Business _____

Business Contact Phone such as boss _____

Other Info _____

Attention Medical Personnel: I have an Advance Directive/Living Will.

_____
Signature

Please consult my document and/or my Power of Attorney in an emergency. My representative is:

Name _____

Address _____

Phone _____

Attention Medical Personnel: My blood type ____.

My allergies:_____ _____

Daily Medications: _____
_____

Epileptic__ Diabetic__ Asthma__ Other_____
_____

Primary Care Physician _____

Phone _____

Attention Medical Personnel:

Contacts to obtain a copy of my Advance Directive.

Name of Agent/Durable Medical Power of Attorney
_____
Phone _____
Name of Alternative Agent/Durable Medical Power of Attorney
_____
Phone _____
Name _____
       Phone

Attention Medical Personnel:

My name: _____

SSN or D/L _____ DOB _____

Insurance Carrier & Number _____

Place of Business _____

Business Contact Phone such as boss _____

Other Info _____

Attention Medical Personnel: I have an Advance Directive/Living Will.

_____
Signature

Please consult my document and/or my Power of Attorney in an emergency. My representative is:

Name _____

Address _____

Phone _____

Attention Medical Personnel: My blood type ____.

My allergies:_____ _____

Daily Medications: _____
_____

Epileptic__ Diabetic__ Asthma__ Other_____
_____

Primary Care Physician _____

Phone _____

Attention Medical Personnel:

Contacts to obtain a copy of my Advance Directive.

Name of Agent/Durable Medical Power of Attorney
_____
Phone _____
Name of Alternative Agent/Durable Medical Power of Attorney
_____
Phone _____
Name _____
       Phone

Attention Medical Personnel:

My name: _____

SSN or D/L _____ DOB _____

Insurance Carrier & Number _____

Place of Business _____

Business Contact Phone such as boss _____

Other Info _____

Notes Page

Notes Page

Notes Page